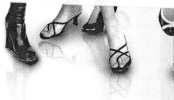

Tommy Orlando

PLAYER'S HANDBOOK

For Men Who Love Women & Sex
(and Want More of Both)

VOLUME 1
Pickup & Seduction Secrets

PLAYER'S HANDBOOK

For Men Who Love Women & Sex (and Want More of Both)

VOLUME 1

Pickup and Seduction Secrets

by
Tommy Orlando

For more information on this series, please visit us on the web at
tommyorlando.com.

KRE, LLC
PO Box 121135
Nashville, TN 37212-1135

CONTENTS

WHEN YOU'RE HOME

INTRODUCTION

Congratulations

You're about to join the ranks of men like me: ordinary guys who have a lot of fun. I meet all kinds of women and have great success. Where? Everywhere. I hook up when I plan on it, and even when I don't. One thing remains the same: I have lots of women around me at all times. They remain my friends forever because I'm a great guy and I know what women want. Women want the same thing guys like us do.

As Sinatra once sang,

> "It's the boys' night out, and they're so romantic,
> I'll give you a clue:
> What the boys are out after,
> The girls are out after too."

Read on and learn the rules that will make you a Player.

Cheers!

Tommy Orlando

A PLAYER DEFINED

A Player is a guy who isn't interested in settling down, but enjoys the company of a woman. In an effort to limit emotions for any one woman, he divides his time among other women at movies, dinner or over coffee. In order to achieve this, A Player must be a planner, a visionary, a communicator, a wit and charming. These skills, natural *and* acquired, help A Player get what he wants—not always sex.

A Player can have coffee with Diane on Tuesday, have sushi with Karen on Thursday, and sleep with Christine on Saturday. And what's the common denominator? Women are present at each event and they like their Player. They may have hopes of a serious relationship, but tolerate this free-spirit who seems oblivious to long-term, romantic love.

These women remain A Player's friend because he shows respect, enjoys the chase, and covers all bases. He may be rejected by women who are hot to marry and perceive his true motives; but for the most part, he enjoys his victories. Women who roll their eyes at a Player are only disappointed that he's beyond their emotional grasp.

The information you're about to read is important for the male gender for many reasons. First, we must combat their strategic books about getting married in 6 months, and finding a guy to support them. We are here to fight fire with fire.

If you apply my information:

→ You will waste less time
→ You will spend less money
→ You will avoid getting hustled
→ You will dodge the female player
→ You will get what you want

Pour yourself a drink, we have work to do.

ABQ: ALWAYS BE QUALIFYING

Player's Rule

ABQ so you don't burn time and money

Always be qualifying. Before I spend precious time and money with someone, I test the waters with simple, qualifying questions so I don't buy $50 in cocktails and four hours later her boyfriend arrives in a Porsche and whisks her away into the evening.

If I want conversation on an airplane, this is not so important; but if I intend to have late night company with someone I met at a restaurant, these questions are critical. Here are the basic qualifiers.

Who Are You Here With?

Sounds like you want to meet her friends, but you really want to determine if she's tethered to a group of nuns or strippers. If you meet her friends and they seem receptive to "the more the merrier" adage, you're in good shape. If her friend(s) seem possessive and try to pull her away, welcome to the uphill battle.

Before you invest time and money in a gal who's going to leave the second her friends snap their fingers, you're better off getting a phone number and taking the high road. Always be as gracious to her friends as you are to her—especially if there's an unattractive friend. If you don't engage her in brief conversation, you'll seem like the divisive one. If you can win her friends' approval, they will be happy for her when you peel her away to the dance floor.

Where Do You Live?

If you're having the time of your life with a woman who will eventually leave the bar and drive eighty miles past road hazards and alcohol checkpoints, she's going to have her guard up. I don't blame her. If she announces she's dreading the drive home, and you're feeling the magic, remind her that your home is hers if she'd rather not take the *dangerous* drive. I have offered many times to sleep on my couch and give her my bed if she decides to stay. If you can get her that far, it can lead to music and Twister.

It's great if she lives around the corner, better if she lives out of state. Why? She doesn't expect you to be her boyfriend, and she's on *vacation*, baby. Something happens to people when they're on the road. When she tells you she's in town visiting a cousin or at a business conference, you can be sure the hormones are in a mild rage. Wherever she's from, ask her if she likes it; whatever her answer, you agree:

Her: "I love Chicago, it's beautiful."
You: "Yeah, I love the Midwest. I like to see the leaves change color."

If she's out of town, she's likely in a hotel and may want company. If she has a long commute, especially with a carload of friends, you may want to cut your losses.

Who Drove?

Wherever she lives, ask how she got to the bar. If she says she's the designated driver, that's going to be difficult. You can't kidnap the bus driver and expect her friends to learn how to work the clutch. Switch gears and go for one of her friends.

If she's alone or one of her friends drove, your chances are better for peeling her off the top of the deck.

What's happening tomorrow?

I fit this in when possible. It's a quick way to gauge how long the night will last. If she tells you she has lunch plans tomorrow, you're golden. If she says she's going to a sunrise mass with her gay neighbor, start looking elsewhere. Nothing kills a mood more than the burden of a big morning the following day. If she's the conscientious type, you can plan on a kiss on the cheek when your Georgia peach turns into a pumpkin.

What do they drink and smoke?

You don't have to ask her this question, just take notice. If she drinks Perrier and asks for twelve limes on the side, make a toast to high maintenance. If she drinks hard liquor with a mixer of some kind, it's cool. If she drinks beer or does a shot, that's real good. Beer is the easiest thing to keep in the house and there's plenty of it around.

If she smokes, that means all she needs is a match and an ashtray at your place and she's content. Let her smoke in the house. Don't sail around the room with a port-a-vac and a can of air freshener. Crack a window and act nonchalant; she wants a drinking buddy, not a housekeeper.

Shifting Gears

Here's a qualifier I've used to sell a girl on moving to a "better" bar: I asked her if she likes "old landmarks—you know, a groovy hang-out that's been there forever and you feel like you're in an old Scorsese movie." She said "yes" and I said "me too."

After we finished the drinks at about the exact same time (I timed it), I acted as if a phenomenal idea popped in my head: "Have you heard of The Iron Horse Tap Room?" I told her it's *exactly* the type of place we were discussing. "Wanna check it out? It's right around the corner?" I added, "Oh what the hell, if you don't like it we'll come right back. I'll leave my tab open (there was no tab), sound like fun?" Bingo. I suggested something I pre-qualified as one of her hot buttons. Ten minutes later we were admiring the iron horse on the wall of The Tap Room.

HOW TO GET A DATE

Player's Rule

Never suggest a night, ask about her schedule

You took a business card from a woman you met at a restaurant a few days ago. You call her because you want to take her out, but you're not sure if she's going to say yes. Here's how to close the deal: instead of asking, "What does Thursday look like on your calendar?" ask her when she has a free night in the next week or two. This works because you don't appear anxious, and you avoid an awkward conversation like this:

You: "What are you doing Wednesday?"
Her: "I have a dinner I need to go to."
You: "How about Thursday?"
Her: "Thursday I'm at a fundraiser."
You: "Oh, what about the weekend?"
Her: "Well, Friday I have plans and Saturday is my parent's anniversary."
You: "Oh, I can call you next week."
Her: "Yeah, call me next week because this week is really crazy."

Please allow me to interpret.

> → Nobody *needs* to go to a dinner
> → Nobody *needs* to be at a fundraiser. People go to fundraisers for the hors d'oeuvres and to meet other singles

→ "Friday plans" means she has a date

→ Her parent's anniversary party—if there is one—is over by nine p.m. and she can be anywhere she wants in fifteen minutes

→ Her week isn't "crazy," unless she's trying to squelch a prison riot—sounds to me like she's eating, partying and screwing through Sunday.

Ask her out like this: "What does your calendar look like in the next week or two?" You know she has one free night. If she still answers the question with a litany of her self-absorbed schedule using words like "audition, Pilate's class, manicure, BMW, and photo shoot," let her go. If you *do* go out with her, you'll have to listen to this nonsense in person—at least on the phone you can watch TV.

Ask about her calendar and let her tell you, "Wednesday looks good." And there you have it. One question, one answer, and you're done. Use sweeping, open-ended questions when choosing a night and you'll save yourself time and embarrassment.

OPENING LINES

Player's Rule

Use common sense when using opening lines

This is a tough one to discuss because it's so circumstantial. Opening lines often relate to something happening at that moment, so I don't have a set of ten great opening lines. I do suggest the following guidelines:

→ They must be sincere
→ They must be relevant

This is discussed in the chapter entitled Be Sincere. Any opening line you employ must be real. If a woman is making a fashion statement with a classic hat, you may tell her, "I want to tell you how much I like your hat." Introduce yourself, ask a good question, and stop talking. Listen.

Avoid deliberate "throw away" lines from Austin Powers' movies.

→ Great legs, what time do they open?
→ Are those reflective pants because I can see my face in them.
→ Somebody call heaven, an angel's missing!

There's nothing wrong with telling a woman, "I think you're very pretty and I'd like to get to know you better." That's honesty *and* sincerity.

If you meet someone and the conversation struggles, bow out gracefully and visit later. She will be more receptive now that you have broken the ice without bending her ear.

An opening line works if it's *relevant*. Here are some events you can build upon and bridge to your opening line:

→ There's a game on TV—"Who's winning?"
→ She's looking at a bar menu—"How's the food here?"
→ It is snowing / raining like crazy—"Have you ever seen weather like this?"
→ It's below zero outside—"Is it cold enough for you today?"
→ Martha Stewart got punched in prison—"Do you feel bad for Martha Stewart?"
→ Donald Trump buys New Jersey—"You think Trump's idea will work?"
→ Your team is in the playoffs—"Do you have plans to go to any of the games?"

These events provide topical entrees to conversation. If you look out the window and comment on the newsworthy weather, a nice person will answer in return. If she doesn't, you've lost very little time and determined that she's not for you.

A final note about opening lines: brace yourself for rejection because it happens. I never invest so much of my ego in an opening line that if she looks at me as if I've got a chicken on my head, I feel bad. I believe in "it's okay if I fail attitude" at this stage of the dance.

REMEMBER HER NAME

Player's Rule

Know her name, use her name

This is critical. When you learn her name, repeat it, memorize it and use it occasionally. Simply say, "Julie? Nice to meet you, Julie, my name is Rob." Burn the name in your short term memory and toss it in the conversation occasionally.

"Where are you from, Julie?" Then later say, "Excuse me, Julie, I need to use the men's room." Dale Carnegie said it best 60 years ago: "The sweetest sound to your ears is the sound of your own first name."

Three ideas if you forget:

1. Listen carefully for someone to address her and then catch her name.
2. Get a friend to introduce themselves and listen for her response.
3. Simply say, "I'm sorry, you told me your name and I've already forgotten it."

Nine times out of ten she's forgotten yours, and you both get one mulligan. Remember her name and you'll be perceived as a man who takes a sincere interest in her as a person.

If her name is unique or interesting, I tell her it is pretty or lovely.

Me: "My name's The Player."

Her: "My name is Sea Breeze."

Me: "Sea Breeze? What a pretty name. And your friend's name is?"

Her: "Sewage."

You: "Sewage? What a lovely name."

You get the point.

BE SINCERE

Player's Rule

Be sincere with your compliments

Women can smell insincerity like roasted garlic. You don't need to make up lies or be insincere with the woman you're with. Find something to like and tell her. If you can't find something you like, you need a new prospect.

Never compliment something they become conscious of and may change—like their laugh. "I love your laugh" will change the frequency and sound of their laughter. Or worse, they'll laugh at things you say that aren't funny. Stick to fixed characteristics.

"You have beautiful hair. I love your long hair. I love your short hair." The key is *believability*. If you try to be charming and compliment the color of a woman's hair and she has frosted tips and a bald spot, she's going to realize you're a bullshitter and be self-conscious about her head the entire evening. *It must be believable.*

If you tell a woman she looks great and she just finished working out, has her hair up, and smells like Karate mats, you'll be flagged as an idiot. She'll apologize for the way she looks and take notice of the pretty girls who made an effort.

Compliment specifics not generalities. "I like your boots" is more effective than "I like the way you dress." "You have beautiful hands" is better than "you are beautiful." "Your left nipple is perfect," might be better than "you have beautiful breasts." A blanket statement is too easy and overwhelming to the listener. Be sincere, be specific, and then be quiet.

COLOGNE

Player's Rule

Less is more

How many times have you shaken hands with someone, and then you smell like his cologne clear to your elbow? Why do amateurs walk around smelling like Bloomingdale's?

I was talking with a couple of gals I knew and, although they smelled great, they were wearing too much of the same perfume. My friends and I were grimacing like we were chopping onions. It's tough to be charming when your eyes are burning. Be sure you don't make that error.

Don't sprits your cologne ten times on your neck and twice down the front of your pants. Guys that smell like lemon rinds, oak barrels, or butterscotch are amateurs. If you even *possess* a bottle of Canoe, Club Man, Old Spice, Aqua Velva, Polo, Chaps, Skin Bracer, or anything that came free with the tie you purchased, stuff a rag in it, light it, and toss it at a rodent. Club Man is in every barbershop in the country and you should wear it if you want to smell like a six dollar haircut.

Use subtle colognes and apply it two hours before you leave the house. If you reek of whatever you wear, you might as well walk around saying, "Hi, I'm Dan, and this is my cologne." They should smell it when you're close, not when you're parking your car.

GUESS MY AGE

Player's Rule

Never play the game

How many times have you had age or weight surface in conversation with women you just met? She says, "I moved here 10 years ago, right after school." You glance to the side and it's clear you're doing math. She asks if you're trying to guess her age, and you deny it. When they try to get you to play the game, resist.

I've stood gazing at wrinkles trying to guess their age, hating myself for playing the game. I'm thinking, "I know she's at least 21 because she's in the bar; she's got to be under 40—" and that's as close as it gets. "Guess my age, my weight, or my cup size" is a losing bet — unless the cup size is a taste test. You will *never* survive the game and emerge victorious.

1. If you guess low, you're a moron and they know you're afraid to take a stand.
2. If you guess correctly, they're disappointed because the game's over and they look their age.
3. If you're over by one year or more, you've bruised their ego and they will feel the sting for two days. Kiss that prospect goodbye.

Tell them you have no idea, tell them you hate games, or change the subject. Wish them a happy birthday, and send them a whipped cream shot, but do not engage them in a game you're sure to lose.

Another danger is "guess my ethnicity." When a girl told me her name was Maria Bella Donna de Benedetti, I said, "Hey, an Italian girl?" She rolled her eyes and asked, "How can you tell?" which is short for "How can you tell, *asshole*?"

On a different occasion, a woman told me her name was Apollonia Snuffoluffogus. I said, "Hey, a Greek girl." She grimaced and said, "No I'm not" which is short for, "No I'm not, *asshole.*" I asked what kind of name it was and she asked me to guess. If it wasn't Greek, I had no flipping idea.

→ Turkish?
→ Sudanese?
→ Eskimo?

She said, "Irish and one quarter Scottish, one quarter Finnish, one quarter Paraguayan, and one quarter Dutch." I didn't really care. I didn't mean to offend her, and I didn't have the heart to tell her that her Finnish grandmother probably banged a Greek guy during spring break around the turn of the century.

Avoid situations you can't win.

WHEN TO BUY A DRINK

Player's Rule

Buying a drink is not the price of admission

"Can I buy you a drink?" is the dumbest of all opening lines. The answer is always yes, and it doesn't mean anything. It doesn't mean she likes you. It doesn't mean she has any interest. It means she's happy to drink your money if that's what you want.

In my early years, I used to buy a drink because I thought it was like holding a door open for a woman or offering her a seat on the subway. It's not a chivalrous thing to do—it's an amateur move. Women have a sense of entitlement. They feel they deserve the drink for wearing their sexy panties. They will not reciprocate. They do not feel obligated to give you a phone number. They may actually *dislike* you, but that doesn't stop them from ordering the eighteen year old scotch. If you want to get her attention, ask if you can buy her a boat.

Buy a drink later if there is progress. After you have some conversation, you've done some qualifying (see chapter ABQ), and she seems receptive while drinking *her* money, then you can offer her a drink. If you're not hot for each other, pretend your cell phone just vibrated in your pocket, ask politely to be excused, and head out the door. When you return, she will be jiggling her ice cubes with an amateur who will buy her next drink.

Beware of women who approach you with an empty glass, they only think your *wallet's* cute. Be a man and look her in the eyes when speaking, not at her glass. If you decide that, drink or not, she's good to go, then you may offer. When you order her drink, tell the bartender that she'll have another. Women love a man that takes control—but you don't need to fill every empty glass. It's a sucker's mission to finance the good times of freeloaders.

HER BIRTHDAY

Player's Rule

Your odds are always good on her birthday

Women love their birthday. They may shrug it off and complain about aging one full year, but they *love* their birthday. Some women openly share that they have a birthday *week*. Some women go out Wednesday through Sunday just to accommodate their friends' schedules and ensure they wring every last drop of celebration out of the occasion. They love the spotlight, and the last thing they want is to be alone.

When you meet a pile of gals who are festive and sharing in laughter, shots and cake, your task is to honor the occasion. The birthday spirit is as strong as Spring Break—all the girls are good to go. The candle isn't the only thing they want to blow. They want kisses, hugs, and an honorary mention every five minutes. Later, they want to be reminded they're a woman. Whatever their taste, it's like a Chinese dinner: it ain't over until they get their cookies.

Address the festivities with renewed confidence that, not only does the birthday girl want attention, but her friends' hormones are flying around the room like a swarm of locusts. They're a rock band: the lead singer gets all the attention, but the drummer some, too. If you can't make it with this crew, it wasn't in the cards.

HER CAREER

Player's Rule

Don't ask, because you don't care

People think careers are a great way to stimulate conversation. No they're not. Most people are self-conscious about what they do and say "food logistics engineer" when they're a waitress. You feign interest trying to avoid glancing at her boobs. Before you kiss her, do you really care how she makes ends meet?

If career comes up in conversation, let her talk about her career and nod your head optimistically at the value and integrity of her chosen career, and try not to look at her boobs. If she asks about your career, keep it short and sweet and down-play it. I don't care if you're an astronaut, mention your career dismissively, and try not to look at her boobs. If you give her tremendous details, you're protesting too much, and she's not listening anyway. She's nodding her head optimistically at the value and integrity of your chosen career as she tries to avoid glancing at her boobs.

I heard a guy tell a group of people, "I essentially market and distribute chemical kits around the world that are used primarily for testing everything from hormones in cows to the safety of the water we drink. We research, test, manufacture, and distribute our patented products to seven different countries. We're privately held now, but expect to put together an IPO in six months that will raise capital and make us the largest" *whatever the fuck blah blah blah!* It doesn't matter what follows, because everybody else is trying to get a peek at her boobs. I heard a guy say he's a producer when he actually works in the produce department at Food Emporium—where he sells melons that look a lot like her boobs.

I've dated PhD's, dancers, attorneys, actresses, dog breeders and an employee from Blockbuster. They were all great women. Some make money, some keep trying, some don't care, some have great boobs, and some are floundering in a sea of dirty martinis. God bless them all. A career doesn't define the person, so avoid giving her the feeling of being qualified.

LISTEN

Player's Rule

You must practice dynamic listening

This rule applies to more intimate settings like dates or one-on-one chatter, not when you address a sea of girls at a beach party.

Women love to talk, and they love it more if you're a good listener. Women are about sharing, venting, and the catharsis of self-expression. You need to close your pie hole and give her that freedom.

Women don't want you to just listen and retain. They want *physical signs* that you are listening. If you glance at the TV, even if you catch every word and detail of her story, you lose points. You must show that you are *physically engaged* in her anecdotes.

This is where body language plays a key role. You must turn your shoulders her direction, make intermittent eye contact and nod your head when appropriate. Smile when she smiles, and encourage her to share more — that's right, *more*. Women don't care how much you know until they know how much you care. Toss in an occasional "Really? Is that right? Wow. What was that like?" As long as they're talking, they feel good and you can't say anything that will blow the deal. The only time I've ever said anything stupid is when I was talking.

I was at a fundraiser speaking to a nice looking woman and she said she was a Vegetarian. I wasn't really listening so I said, "Wow, sounds like you take care of yourself." And it continued like this:

"I do okay," she replied. "Once I got the practice up
    and running."
"Takes practice to eat broccoli?" I kidded.
"What?"
"You said eating right takes practice."
"No I didn't."
"You said you practice something and I said
    eating broccoli."
"Excuse me?"

This continued for another annoying minute until I realized she said *veterinarian*. We were two sentences away from asking, "What the fuck are you talking about?" I once thought a woman told me she was a penis, but later realized she played the piano.

Listening is your job. If you let a woman share her feelings, you will know how to appeal to her hot buttons. If she's an obvious humanitarian, give the homeless guy a couple of bucks on the way to your car. If she's spiritual, pour her green tea the next morning. You will know what to do based on the information you gathered using dynamic listening skills.

EVERYTHING IS CLOSE

Player's Rule

Nothing is complicated and everything is close

Logistics must be simple. As comedian Kip Addotta says, "If I could change the world, I would make everything just around the corner and on the right hand side of the street." If you call a girlfriend when you're out having a good time, and you want her to join you, tell her she's only a few minutes away—especially if she's never heard of the place.

Women don't like to drive. It means they have to rush to get ready and then fool with the car, the clutch, and the cruelest of all unusual punishments: park and pay in valet. Keep everything real simple.

As far as she knows, you just arrived at the bar. This eliminates her fear of joining you as you pay your check and leave for the next bar. Tell her to take her time, you just got there, and you have a barstool for her if she wants it.

If she asks where the place is, tell her it's down the street, even if the street is Route 66. Actually, *you must be honest*. You shouldn't cajole a woman into an evening of traffic in the Holland Tunnel or a wild goose chase out to the Hinterlands. She'll never speak to you again—but make the somewhat simple seem *very* simple. Have a carefree attitude because it's catching. If you lower your voice and give directions using words like "fork, jug handle, dogleg, off-ramp, rotary, bridge, access road, side street, alley, and toll booth," she'll reach for her pistol. If we believe the earth is somewhat close to the sun, you're close to wherever she is when she answers her phone.

WATCH THE CLOCK

Player's Rule

Always be secretly aware of the time

Getting what you want is all about timing. You have to say the right thing at the right time. If you try to close the deal one minute before she thinks you've earned it, it's over. If you drag your feet and wait too long, the attraction loses its momentum. Be aware of the time like a fighter pilot is aware of his flight coordinates.

If you wear a watch or use your cell phone as your time piece, make an occasional glance *unbeknownst* to her. You never want to get caught worrying about the time. It makes people curious or suspicious. You don't want to look like you're trying to catch a train or time your next medication; it's like Vegas: the attitude is upbeat, the action is everywhere, and there's a general disregard for time when you're having fun. At least that's how you want it to appear.

The reality is there are several ways in which time affects your strategy. What time do you need to get your car out of valet? What time do they tow cars off the street? When is last call? When do they turn up the lights at the bar? When does the sun rise? What time does the liquor store close? When do the trains stop running? If you get burned because you missed a "deadline," all your efforts fly out the window. Let's look at a few scenarios.

Last call is *not* an invitation to begin chapter two somewhere else—unless she's a fan of speakeasies or underground raves in shady warehouses. Once you hear the bartender indicate last call, beware for whom the bell tolls, it tolls for thee. The bar is rushed by people who want another three for the road, and people who want to close their tab, both of which overwhelm the bartender. Now you're fifteen minutes away from getting your check.

I was having a great time at a bar in New York City with a pretty, dark-haired Irish girl. Van Morrison was singing a ballad from the jukebox and rain fell softly on Columbus Avenue. I lost track of time and soon it was last call. We didn't need cocktails so we continued mumbling in the din of the bar.

Suddenly, the jukebox went silent and spotlights around the bar burned brightly. It was like having cocktails in a racquetball court. We squinted at each other and quickly inventoried the freckles, razor burn and other imperfections. The bar was littered with napkins and swizzle sticks. I tried to get out of there in order to salvage the mood.

Be aware of how much time you have left in order to close the deal. Leave the room or advance the game before the fat lady sings, and you can sustain the illusion that the evening is still rolling.

MARRIED WOMEN

Player's Rule

The chase is reserved for single women

I've been there many times. I'm in flirt mode and start talking before I check for a ring on her finger. The vibe is strong but then their wedding ring flashes at me like the paparazzi. It takes discipline, but my experience says let her go.

Part of my decision is karma; the other is for my personal safety. When you decide to settle down, you wouldn't want others to see your wife as fair game, so take the high road and leave married people with their spouses. Stay away from women who want some loving before their husband returns from a hunting trip—he may be hunting her last boyfriend.

In terms of safety, let me share a story. I went out with a thirty year-old woman who failed to tell me she was married-but-having-problems and left the ring at home that day. We boink and a week later I get a phone call from her husband. He found my number on her history of dialed calls on her cell phone. He questioned her, she buckled on the witness stand, and he did some speed dialing.

Meanwhile, I'm at home watching David Letterman and brushing my teeth. My phone rings and I see it's her number. I answered with, "French kisses, this is Johnny speaking, and how may I help you?" I was greeted with, "FUCK YOU

ASSHOLE! YOU A TOUGH GUY? SHOW ME HOW FUCKING TOUGH YOU ARE!" He sounded like he lived in a barn and ate goats. He told me how many different ways he would separate my bones and then told me to go have intercourse with myself in my own rectum.

I pleaded innocent and told him to forget this ever happened. He wasn't ready for friendship or exchanging emails. This was *not* a no harm, no foul discussion. Neither one of us said, "I feel your pain." He promised to one day hand me my teeth and hung up. When my house went bump in the night, I was sure it was him on my roof with a crowbar.

If he had caught us, and decided to spank me with a nine iron, it would be understandable behavior in a court of law. A crime of passion when spouses cheat is a breeze for a jury: the women feel you deserve it, and the men would have upgraded to their titanium driver. This was bad and it was an *accident*. Don't make this mistake.

GETTING HER PHONE NUMBER

Player's Rule

When you have no choice, get her cell phone

This strategy is a bit of a cheat, but it's fool proof. Use it at your own risk.

Sometimes you're talking to a woman and other people are within ear-shot or her protective friends have formed a semi-circle and have been cock-blocking for the last hour. You have great rapport with this woman and it's obvious you would have fun together another time. What do you do? You don't want to sound cheesy asking for her number. Her girlfriends will tell her to get *your* card and maybe *she'll* call. Okay, now all bets are off.

Here's what to say: "Lisa, do you get reception in here?" Let her look at her phone while you furrow your brow at your poor reception. She will say something like, "Yeah, I've almost got a full signal." Ask, "What service do you have?" What ever she says, you have the competitor. Now look at your phone shaking your head "no" and curse the other service. Then ask, "Could I call my office voicemail for just a quick second? It's a local call."

This is a no-brainer for her because she likely has 5,000 free minutes a month for local and long distance. I've never had anybody say no. You need to get this done quickly while her girlfriends are cackling somewhere else.

When you get her phone, call your cell phone. Let it vibrate until voicemail picks up and then hang up. Tell her you're getting a busy signal which is "weird." Now what do you have? Her number stored in your history of incoming calls. Sweet. Now change the subject: "You know Ford is coming out with a new sport utility vehicle?"

Later, when you're out of sight, store the number under her name and you have no worries. You're free from the beady-eyed scrutiny of her girlfriends, and it's faster than getting a cocktail napkin and locating a pen.

Here's the risk: when you surprise her with a phone call, she'll ask, "Hey, how'd you get my number?" Sometimes you can humor your way out of it by saying, "a little birdie gave it to me." And then change the subject: "Where are you right now?"

I've had women baffled, flattered, or violated that I found a clever way to get their number. If she doesn't have a sense of humor about it, it's a sign that you were sure to do something else she would find offensive.

BOOTY CALLS

Player's Rule

Never sound desperate

These are tricky, especially after a few cocktails. Be aware of how transparent a booty call is. Women forgive us for the stupidity and glaring desperation of a late night call after half a dozen cocktails. We are not clever. We are not fooling anybody. We are no longer smooth at this point in the evening; they only let us think we are.

Remember this:

1. The girl you call realizes that she wasn't your first pick for the evening agenda
2. The girl you call realizes you're drunk
3. The girl you call realizes that she may have been the fourth number dialed

That being said, let's focus on minimizing the scope of our foolishness.

Beware of the rambling booty call. It sounds like this:

"Hey Debbie, it's me. What's happening, hot stuff? I'm here at some bar with my buddies and I'm gonna leave soon—gonna get the fuck outa here—any who—where *are* you? PICK UP THE PHONE!—just kidding, I know it's your voicemail—any who, I'm gonna be heading back soon and I would *love* to see you tonight if you just wanna hang out, or just chill or whatever—it's up to you; but (belch) oops, let me get the fuck outa here and I'll *definitely* call you in a little bit, okay? This is Bill by the way. Okay. Talk to you then. Bye, babe. This is Bill. Okay, bye."

She heard three things in the message:

1. "I'm drunk"
2. "I'm a caveman"
3. "I'm horny"

There's only one reason why she's going to return your call and come over later:

1. She's drunk
2. She likes cavemen
3. She's horny

Fortunately, women are as bad as men, and they will tolerate this at least for a while. Pretty soon she wants to be asked out on a regular date, she prefers you sober, she'll want you to shower, and she won't want sex, she'll want to make love.

Here's how to avoid the voicemail that wears its very own dunce cap:

1. Call her before you see double
2. Tell her you have terrible cell phone reception
3. Tell her you're at dinner and would love to see her later

If she's sober and you're slurring, it can be a put off, unless she thinks drooling and farting is charming. Get the message to her before your wheels fall off.

Tell her you have terrible phone reception so you can buy yourself some time. If she calls back and you're tossing olives down Angela's cleavage, you have a few moments to finish the game.

If you find yourself pursuing a better offer, call her and tell her you're home and almost asleep. If you want to ensure that she doesn't come over, tell her you think you ate a bad oyster and your stomach's in a tizzy; or, don't answer at all and tell her you came home and crashed on the couch watching M*A*S*H.

Finally, never answer the phone unless the incoming number shows on your cell phone. It's too risky. The wrong girl will call at the wrong time and hear the wrong voice in the background, and you'll be in trouble. If the call's important they will leave a message and you can check it after you finish with Angela.

BREATH MINTS

Player's Rule

Keep some kind of breath freshener with you at all times

This doesn't mean you should always have a mint in your mouth. It's not Halloween. This rule suggests you should always have the *option* for better breath.

Pay attention smokers: to the nonsmoker your breath smells like Uncle Frank after a cigar smoothie. Some women are okay with it, but play it safe and carry a few mints. Food is a consideration as well. One Caesar salad or a crock of onion soup and you smell like a garbage bin in August to other innocent victims.

→ Buy small mints with an adult name. Avoid names like "Spearmint Explosion!" or "Peppermint Frenzy!" No Pez dispensers or anything in the shape of animals. Never carry a super-sized box of Altoids that rattle with your every step. Unless you save the comic strip in your gum, grow the fuck up.

Keep the flavor adult as well. Avoid flavors like

→ Banana split
→ Coconut Breeze
→ Cannelloni de Roma

Keep it in your mouth tucked between your cheek and gum. It will last 30 minutes or more and it helps two ways: you will have greater confidence and she will appreciate your minty breath.

BLOCKING

Player's Rule

Blocking is for amateurs

Sometimes men try to win the attention and approval of women by being clever in their presence or physically vying for their attention. There is nothing wrong with cleverness, but a witticism at a friend's expense is a bad move. Chasing women is not a game of physically shouldering out the competition.

People are attracted to you because of your optimism, your smile and your attitude. The cynic always sits alone. Avoid taking digs at your pals with comments like, "What does he know, he thinks Mt. Rushmore's a natural rock formation;" or, "You're talking to a guy who buys his shirts at the liquor store;" or, "Nice suit, Tom, do they make it in your size?"

Sure, people will giggle, but it creates an uncomfortable tension. You can win friends faster by paying those around you compliments, not criticisms. It's a cheap shot to make time with a woman ahead of your cronies by blurting mean-spirited one-liners.

If you're with a group of buddies and one of your friends is making time with a woman, leave him alone. It's dirty pool to wait for him to tie his shoe so you can lean in with a business card. If he's a friend, The Player's Code disapproves of hiding in the ladies room so you can introduce yourself.

It's okay to eventually meet them, but it must be aboveboard. Introduce yourself publicly. If a friend has time and money invested in a woman, it's unfair to wedge your way in and begin a subtle game of footsy while he orders her a drink. A Player relies on other methods of winning approval.

I remember a night with my pals (let's call them Moe, Larry and Curly) when the blocking was in full bloom and, naturally, it backfired.

Moe was talking to a girl on a barstool with his hand on her knee. Larry walks up and attempts to impress her by insulting the bartender he's know for years. "Hey dickhead, when you get a chance, how about two more?" and "Hey dip shit, I said a lemon."

Then along came Curly. He approached from the rear and started massaging her shoulders. Moe rambled on about the Bears' pre-season while Larry continued to delight in his insulting orders which had progressed to "pencil-neck" and "snaggletooth." After ten minutes, Moe had rubbed her into a blister, Larry ran low on insults, and she grabbed her purse and left. It was the Nature Channel personified with the male species strutting and dancing in circles. Unless you're a gorilla or a pheasant, this never pays off.

SISTERS

Player's Rule

You won't get far with sisters

You may know of an exception to this Player's rule, but by and large, sisters mean no dice.

If you and your buddy meet sisters, you'll find they look out for each others' best interests and they hesitate to be themselves in front of each other:

→ "Sheila! I didn't know you smoke!"
→ "Hey, where's my sister going?!"
→ "Stop lifting my sister's skirt!"
→ "No, she's *not* doing another shot of Jack Daniels!"
→ "You can spank me, but not in front of my sister!"
→ "Debbie, you need to fix the button on your shirt."
→ Untie my fucking sister!"

Soon, the sisters with tattoos of the devil on their pelvis seem subdued and pure. Amber, the local stripper, is now rather Pollyanna-ish. Why? Because sisters don't like to see sisters act naughty.

There are some exceptions and I've seen them, but generally the fun takes place outside of the family.

THE TRUTH ABOUT COWORKERS

Player's Rule

Nobody can keep a secret

"Let's keep this under our hat" is one of the least employed promises. The truth about coworkers is simple: if you engage in romance, it's always risky and everybody talks.

Imagine the complexity of your day when you're sleeping with a coworker. Pretty soon you begin to dress for *her*. You work hard at *not* flirting or you feign disinterest which only adds to the sexual tension. You spend time impressing her. You grip your briefcase on the side like a football, not using the handle; you type like Elton John at a piano; you make audible grunting noises when using the paper cutter. After a while you get tired of playing the game and now you're stuck with old baggage at the office all day. If you get caught on the phone speaking to another woman, she'll roll her eyes and tell other co-workers that you're A Player.

Additionally, the two of you are not the only ones who know about this. Men talk when they drink, women talk when they pee. Somehow she leaked it to a friend who mentioned it at the company shuffleboard party. Even you told a few friends.

There are approximately 4,568,070 good looking women in the U.S. (give or take 518). Two of them work in your office and you can't resist. I understand. But when you weigh the drama, passion, and comedy against the one night you had with her for an hour of drama, passion and comedy, is it really worth it?

HIGHLIGHTING YOUR IMPERFECTIONS

Player's Rule

Never draw attention to your imperfections

Sometimes men try to get a laugh or charm their way to acceptance by using self-deprecating humor. This is okay to a point. If you shine too much light on one of your faults, it grows in the minds of the listeners.

Recently, I was out with the guys at a great bar. A pretty girl walked in, hung her coat beside me and went to the bar to wait for a girlfriend. We acknowledged each other and I asked her to join us. She came over and soon we were all friends.

She later told us a story about why she doesn't wear earrings: she said she has low-hanging lobes. I didn't notice but when she turned her head and began tugging on one of her ear lobes, they were the size of thumbs. I couldn't listen to her stories because I was distracted by the wiggling lobes that swung each time she looked a different direction. I pictured her face on the cover of National Geographic.

The following are lines I've collected over the years and actually heard people use in an attempt to establish rapport:

→ After being offered a light beer: "C'mon, look at me! Do I look like I drink diet anything?" And he patted his belly like a woman in her 7th month of pregnancy.

→ Commenting on a guy with a full head of hair: "I had hair like him once. I'm starting to look like Homer Simpson." He wasn't even close to bald but the tiny area that was thinning now glared through the bar.

→ A woman complimented a friend and said she's showing beautiful cleavage: "Oh please, these two shot glasses?" And for the rest of us her boobs all but disappeared.

I → actually heard a festive drunk say, "What do I care—I gotta small pecker, what am I gonna do?!" And he laughed seeking approval. Unless you want women picturing a wine cork in your pants, steer clear of this wizardry.

If you must use self-deprecating humor, limit it to

- → I'm always late
- → I'm the worst speller
- → Math isn't my strength
- → I'm terrible at remembering first names
- → I'm a sweet tooth

Leave out the physical because we see what we need to see, and we don't need our imaginations emboldened by your comments.

FIGHTS

Player's Rule

It's rarely worth the effort

Fights are avoidable. If you're defending your honor or just caught a guy with his hand in your back pocket, give him an elbow to the neck. If a guy is looking at your woman, bats his eyes at her, or is talking to her when you return from the bathroom, be cool. That's the price of having a good looking woman with you.

This is not your test, it's hers. A woman who's with you on a date owes you the respect of her undivided attention. She should turn her shoulder to the competition, not sit on his knee. If she engages another guy in conversation, laughs hysterically at his jokes or puts her hand on his forearm when talking, find a bartender and whisper "check please." I'm not the jealous type, but I'm also not there to feed her food and liquor while she works the room. This is where you cut the date so short the car arrives before the check and you start dialing for the next date with your free hand.

If you just met someone and the same scenario happens, you don't have the same claim to her time and attention. Just because you've spent the last ten minutes debating whether or not fellatio counts as sex, doesn't mean the girl's your property. Once she downs your drink she's a free agent. Punching a guy in the face for hitting on this village bar fly is out of line and dangerous. If you win the fight, you're an asshole that has just burned a bridge at one of your hangouts—and it doesn't mean she's going home with you.

If you lose the fight, it's a double disgrace. You spent a few bucks and a few minutes with a girl and tried to impress her with your short temper. Now the barstools are on the floor and you're holding what's left of your shirt. Enjoy the ride home. You can and should avoid challenging a drunk. Fights are a mood kill, not an aphrodisiac.

HUMOR

Player's Rule

Never tell a joke

You've never seen a woman look around the bar and ask, "Hey, you guys know any good jokes?" Jokes rarely work and it's usually the alcohol that makes them mildly amusing. Jokes wear people out; however, a sense of humor is always welcomed. Have the balls to use your natural, God-given sense of humor.

A joke obligates the listener to perform at the end of your punch line. They must smile and point at the joke teller. Nine times out of ten, you never get the laugh you hoped for. You hear a few groaner giggles and mumbles. Somebody yells "ba-dump-dump." Another says "Don't quit your day job." And if the joke is long, double mistake! Never tell a joke that involves accents, props or visuals. People who tell jokes that require intermission and a concession stand should be banished. If you *must* tell a joke it should take less than ten seconds.

If you blow the joke you look like a circus clown without the cute outfit. You ask, "Can bankers earmark money for a hearing aid?" They say "that's funny"—a sign that it's not.

And no magic tricks. Don't pull out the silk handkerchief, the "floating dollar," pull a bra from a hardboiled egg, or any other stocking stuffer intended for children ages 5-8. People hire magicians at children's birthday parties. Don't embarrass yourself. Leave the deck of cards, the walnut shells and Mexican jumping beans at home.

HOW TO DRIVE

Player's Rule

Your car is for transportation, it's not a recording studio

Let's start outside the car. Open the door for her the first time, but never after that. They'll think you watch too many etiquette videos. I believe in the old expression, "When a man opens a car door for a woman, it's either a brand new car, or a brand new woman." Unless you want to look like Greg Brady in his dad's car, don't overdo opening the door — it even makes them uncomfortable. A guy that does this all the time is hiding something. You're her date, not a valet.

When driving, keep your hands on the wheel. Absolutely no air guitar, no air cymbals, no drums on the dashboard, and don't point the fucking invisible microphone in her direction. You are there to get to your destination efficiently and safely, not to entertain her with the first two lines of a song, and then every third word. Save it for karaoke.

The interior of your car should not smell like a pine tree, tangerines, or talcum powder. Clean the car, keep it clean, and don't eat, shave, or drink in the car. Nothing turns off a woman more than a ride in a car with a sticky console, and an emergency brake cluttered with crumbs, French fries and two pennies you couldn't reach. Your car is an extension of your personality and overall hygiene. Don't lose the deal over something simple like a car that looks like a college dorm.

Don't stop at green lights that may turn yellow any second, but don't blow every frigging yellow light. If she has to put her hand on the dashboard more than twice when you're driving, she'll have the runs by the time you get back to the house. Drive like a normal guy. Use this time to converse and listen (See Listen chapter.)

AIRPLANES

Player's Rule

If you screw up you can't leave

If you're A Player, you travel occasionally by plane. You may go to Vegas for a weekend, Chicago for the big convention, or to Kansas to visit Auntie Em. A Player knows no boundaries and always has their antennae extended for the next opportunity. If opportunities arise anywhere, you must be prepared everywhere.

Dress Code

Shakespeare said it's the clothes that make the man, so dress appropriately. Some people think travel should be comfortable so they wear sweats and a t-shirt that looks like it was pulled from the washer and worn damp to the airport. If you think women are attracted to five bucks worth of clothing, go for it. A shopping bag isn't luggage. And unless you're a gymnast, leave the tank top for the monkey bars. Err on the side of smart but casual.

Seating

I always take an aisle seat so I can take a leak without the permission of three people on their laptops, and I have the added value of conversing with a passerby. Conversation is initiated only after I have sized up the situation. Never become the bore who expects dialogue from wheels-up until the next gate.

When you're seated and waiting for someone to fill the empty seat beside you, do not comment on the person who arrives, man or woman. If it's a man, don't say, "Well, I had my hopes up for a young blonde." And if *it is* a young blonde who asks if she can squeeze in, the answer is not, "abso-friggin-lutely" or "you betcher bippy." It kills the suspense of what you are thinking.

Be polite as you glance up from the book you're pretending to read. I carry a copy of *How to make your Third Million.*

Chivalry
Airplanes offer a number of ways you can be a good guy and help a damsel in distress:

- → Help her with luggage in the overhead compartment
- → Allow her to use the lavatory first
- → Offer her your bag of 6 peanuts that comes with your 2 ounce Pepsi

Making conversation can be a bit tricky. Some women are okay because it passes the time and they don't have much of a choice. Others (like me), are reluctant to make eye contact because it opens doors to rapport that are tough to close. How do you switch from dialogue to silence unless you close your eyes and wear headphones?

On the other hand, I've had friends that have landed a hot woman they met on a plane—some even close the deal on the plane and join the "mile-high" club after half a Pepsi and two peanuts.

If you can't work your magic on the plane, you have one final shot: baggage claim. If you've already flirted with someone on the plane and then lost track of them, you can rest assured she's checked a bag and will be at the same baggage claim carousel ten minutes after you arrive at the gate. If you approach her there, you'll need to do some quick qualifying so you don't carry her bag to the curb where her sharply dressed mobster friend is waiting in his Lincoln.

LIGHTING

Player's Rule

Find warm lighting and adjust it before you leave for the evening

Lighting is the world you create when you are together. It affects how you feel about each other when you are out. I frequent bars and restaurants with amber bulbs and red lampshades because it's warm and cozy and everybody looks good. The mood is intimate long before you get a chance to be. If you go to a brasserie with glaring white lights, you might as well go for ice cream at Baskin Robbins.

Have good lighting at your house. If you have bright lights and need them for whatever reason, have a second set of Player lights. Monica Lewinsky is living proof that President Clinton had a dimmer switch in the Oval Office. Soft, pink light bulbs are great, even the amber bulb in the corner is like a small fireplace—but don't make the living room look like a lava lamp because that may backfire. There's a fine line between *A Player's Den* and a *Den of Iniquity*. They shouldn't be leery of sitting on the couch in a skirt.

Before you leave the house for the night, adjust the lighting. Nothing kills a mood faster than leaving a romantic place and returning home to what looks like the frozen food aisle. If you need to squint when you get home, you've made a tactical error. And it's an amateur move to get on your knees and plug in "the cool lamps," dim the overheads, and try to unscrew hot light bulbs while she stands there holding her purse. She'll think you're working much too hard and thoughts of, "Relax pal, it may not go that far," sail through her head.

MUSIC

Player's Rule

Create a play list of songs
that create your desired mood

If you're in your home, music is as critical as lighting (see Lighting chapter). Music affects mood, so choose music that creates the mood for your desired outcome and cue it up for your return. If you return home to The Lawrence Welk Orchestra and have to drop to your knees in a suit to find jewel cases and out-of-order CD's, you've made a tactical error.

I'll leave the music selection up to you, with a few caveats: avoid deliberate let's-get-laid music. The throaty Barry White stuff worked in the 70's but today it's worse than just throwback. The Bee Gee's are throwback. Barry White is a bit over the top as he whispers, "Oh baby, take off that brassiere, my dear." Keep the music selections conducive to what you want and avoid the cheesy stuff. If you both want to dance, play dance music. If you want to talk, play music that lends itself to good conversation, not Emminem's rants about killing his mother. If you're studying for a final exam, try one of the Bach Sonatas.

It's best to create a mix of tunes you like. Never play one continuous band for two reasons: 1) they shift from fast to slow and you may want it all one way or the other; and 2) too much of the same thing can backfire. Play a variety of music and push the repeat button so the CD's are on continuous loop. It's a mood kill when the music stops and you're in the bathroom flushing and blowing your nose.

If you recognize the music starts to repeat, play another compilation. Don't ask her what she likes, you may not have anything even close, and you will seem incompatible.

WHEN TO CANDLE

Player's Rule

Less is more and be safe

Candles are great, but your home should not look like the vestibule of St. Patrick's Cathedral or a Romanian séance. Only women take twenty minutes to light every flipping candle they own. One or two is fine.

Use one of those long lighters that can light the deepest of candles. It's an amateur move to take regular matches and burn your fingers three times before you have a success. Have the right tools and light a couple of candles, but keep an eye on them.

I've had three mishaps:

> → I awoke the next day to find three candles burned to the nub and a circle of wax the size of a trashcan lid all over my dining room table.

> → I placed candles on the mantle above the fireplace and lost track of details, only to find a wax stalactite drooling all over my fireplace screen.

> → I left an aromatherapy candle on the back of my toilet and my date—who had long, curly hair almost to her waist—sat down, flipped her hair back over the candle and didn't notice what was happening until she saw ashes flying around the bathroom. She screamed bloody murder and I came running.

When she unlocked the door, I was overcome by the stench of burning hair. In the end, she didn't lose that much hair; I apologized and let her take a three-hour shower while I watched Sports Center.

My date was a great sport about it once she realized things were okay. I thought about her everyday that week — it took that long to get the smell out of the house.

SUPPLIES

Player's Rule

A Player's house is not a home without the right supplies

If you plan to entertain, you must have the basic ingredients. If you fail in this category, it's impossible to be cool. You'll never charm a woman if all you can offer is Blueberry Liqueur or a tall glass of Cinnamon Schnapps. You can survive the evening, but they may not return.

Basic ingredients include Vodka, Tequila, White Wine and a few options for mixers: cranberry, soda, tonic water. Have it in the house but not in large bottles. Don't make a Martini with a huge bottle of vodka you bought at Sam's Club with handles on both sides. If you need to embrace the bottle in order to pour it, you need to scale down the size.

Avoid the Bart Simpson bottle opener, and other gimmicks. Women take notice of these accoutrements. You got her to the one-yard line; don't blow it by dropping a lime on the floor, wiping it on your shirt and putting it in her drink.

A friend of mine had a few people over and served cocktails in red plastic cups. Unless there's a keg on ice in your bathtub, I wouldn't do that. He then used his fingers to fish out a maraschino cherry and put it in a cocktail glass he washed from the sink. We felt like we needed tetanus shots.

Here are a few things to avoid when hosting a woman:

→ Don't snap bottle caps across the living room
→ Rose's Lime Juice is not a shot
→ Don't serve drinks with a striped straw unless you've made chocolate malts
→ Don't stir a cocktail with a fork
→ If your drink is too strong, don't spit it back in the glass
→ I don't drink out of a container that has the name of a bar, sports team, or dumb statements like, "My grandmother went to a swingers' club and all I got was this stupid glass."

Limes and lemons are inexpensive and nice touches when serving cocktails. Have plenty of ice. Buy a wine opener that works and use appropriate glasses. You can't pour champagne in a beer mug. Get your hands on the right supplies and your presentation will improve.

CASH & CONDOMS

Player's Rule

Always have plenty of cash and condoms

One of the worst errands to run when you're with a woman is for cash or condoms. I don't like to stop anywhere if I can help it whether I'm in a taxi or my own car.

If you stop for cash, that tells her you're a dolt who pulls out twenty dollars at a time from the cash machine, and when you spend it, you go back for another twenty. If you're a real dolt, you insist on using the cash machine that's part of your bank network so you can avoid the whopping one dollar charge. Avoid this by having a little extra cash on you when you're out. I carry plenty of just-in-case money and use a credit card if I don't want to burn the cash.

If you must stop for condoms, it tells her one of three things:

1. You never get laid so this is a big event
2. You always get laid and you go through condoms like Q-Tips
3. You never use condoms but it might be safer with a girl like her

Have a condom with you in case you go to her place. It's responsible and you never want a girl to tell you she'll sleep with you "if you have a condom" and you don't. I've stood there with my pants around my ankles wondering if wrapping it in something will do the trick—amateur move.

Once I stopped for condoms and told her I was buying margarita mix. I parked the car, entered the small Korean market, got the mix and whispered for a pack of condoms. He put them on the counter and then decided to change the receipt tape at the register. A line formed behind me and the world knew I was thirsty and horny. As I tapped my fingers on the counter, she walks in and tells me to buy ice because her icemaker is broken. She sees the little party I have planned and yells "bad boy!" She had a sense of humor but it did reveal my true intentions on the counter in plain Korean and English.

If you're at your house and she asks if you have a condom, tell her you think so, and then look around a bit. Don't go into the garage and don't lean over and pull them from the drawer like a Musketeer; the former says amateur, the latter says pro. Women want men who are a bit savvy at the game of Playing, not Ph.D.'s.

It happened to me at a woman's house. We were rolling around and she asked if I had a condom with me. I pretended I wasn't sure and she said, "That's okay, I have one here." She reached over to the nightstand and lifted an accordion of continuous feed foil condoms. The words "Lubricated, Reservoir, Ribbed, Ultra and Sensitive" flashed before my eyes. I felt this girl should have a turnstile installed in her doorway. I imagined that these sheets weren't only warm, but possibly damp.

Nobody, unless she's a pro, wants irrefutable evidence that you're A Player. Even if you think *she* gets around, you don't want to see her kicking a pair of boxer shorts under her bed or hiding the gun a guy left behind. Keep the obvious in the implied category, down-play your competency and experience and you'll give each other the respect of an evening that means something.

HOTEL ROOMS

Player's Rule

Your hotel room should inspire your craft

Hotels are fun because you have access to room service and, even if she lives a mile away, she feels like she's on vacation. If you have plans with a woman while staying at a hotel, you may want her back to your room later. Keep the room clean and conducive to the party:

→ Read the chapter on Lighting for lighting ideas
→ Read the chapter on Music for music etiquette (With laptops and iPods, your music choices can follow you everywhere).
→ Read the chapter on Snooping and remember that she's going to snoop

The Room

If you know you'll be having a guest, choose a room that reflects your sophistication. If your room is tiny and on the ground floor with a panoramic view of the air conditioning system, you'd better have a perfect score with the other Player's Rules.

You don't need to blow big money on a suite, but get a higher floor, ask about the view (overlooking the river or the nuclear plant?), and see if the front desk is in the mood for an upgrade. A little space goes a long way.

Room Prep

After I shower and get ready, I always ask housekeeping to "turn down the room." This means they will have it cleaned like it was when you checked in, replace towels, fold down the sheets and add some boxed chocolates on the pillow. It's a major mood kill if you skip this step.

A few years ago I asked for turn down service and left the room. Housekeeping never showed and when I returned with the pretty girl in a wonder bra, we were welcomed by a bed that had been slept in, a pile of damp towels, Kleenex floating in the toilet, water on the bathroom tile, my room service tray on the desk, and a pair of boxer shorts on the TV.

I told her to have a seat on the chair near what was left of my chicken dinner. I handed her the remote as if it were a glass of Champagne and shuffled around the room kicking towels and mopping the floor with my boxers.

Finally, I always arrange the wake up call before I leave the room. I've had too many nights cocktailing on the balcony and excusing myself to leave the wakeup call. Nothing kills the present mood more than the reminder that you need to wake up in three hours – might as well walk around in your Spiderman pajamas. If the wakeup call is requested before you leave, you can relax and feign a devil-may-care attitude.

Snooping

She will snoop—you can bank on it. Here's the strategy: leave things you want her to see, hide the things you don't.

You want her to see your vitamins, Wall Street Journal, protein powder, and fancy conditioner with the French name.

Hide your personal lubricant, condoms, anti-gas tablets, Viagra, ear wax stabilizer, and anything for pimples. Put those in the garment bag that's hidden under the bed.

Be a great host and you can charm the thong off anyone.

BLAME IT ON THE HOUSEKEEPER

Player's Rule

What ever the problem, blame it on the housekeeper

If your home is too neat and she calls you a clean-freak, blame it on the housekeeper. Say something like, "Tell me about it, my housekeeper was here twice this week and she cleans everything three times." Housekeeper is better than "maid" and it's a sign of a busy guy with a little extra cash.

If your home is a mess and she says a tornado must have hit it, blame it on your housekeeper: "She takes a vacation every time someone on TV has a baby. She asked for three days off this month and I got lazy."

If you pour her beer in a coffee cup, tell her your housekeeper is either stealing or breaking all the good glassware. Act nonchalant and change the subject: "I hear Gruyere cheese is getting very expensive."

DRUGS

Player's Rule

Drugs are for amateurs

I'm sure in the sixties and seventies the closing line was "wanna go back and smoke a joint?" It probably worked and that kind of close is okay. I disagree with bartering drugs for sex or using drugs as a way to have your way.

You've seen the swarthy man wearing five rings searching for a girl who would love some cocaine. He couldn't have his way with a monkey if he had a fistful of bananas. You don't need skills if you pay for it with drugs or money.

If you try to get your girl completely loaded and then back to your house you're asking for trouble. Back in college, I held plenty of girls' hair in a pony tail as they swayed over the toilet. Unless you keep a gallon of Miracle Vomit under the sink, be cool with the booze.

If you funnel shots with a girl so she'll follow your lead, that's cheating. A Player can reel a girl out of a church pew ten minutes before her own wedding without the help of Jack Daniels. Moreover, if she's trashed at your house and takes a header down a flight of stairs, you'll have some explaining to do with the police and forensic pathologist; don't get me wrong, cocktails are in abundance at my place late night, but it's not the way I get them there.

Needless to say, these morons who slip things in people's drinks should be in jail. If a guy drinks a shot of tea while he sends a whisky shot to a girl, he should have "pussy" tattooed on his forehead. If you can't use words and charm to get what you want, unfair shortcuts break The Players Code.

GAMES

Player's Rule

Use games to break the ice

Games are fun, especially if you're with a few buddies and their dates. Games are a way to ease the burden of carrying on conversation. Games are a great way to reveal peoples' true nature. There's a quote that suggests you can learn more about a person's true nature in an hour of play than a year of friendship. When fitting, pull out a simple game and start the charm—but it must be the right kind of game.

Games must be *very* simple. If she's had dinner and a glass of wine and soon finds herself learning that Artemis is the daughter of Zeus and Leto, and must lose two elixirs for landing on a blue square, she's going to plan her exit strategy. I don't recommend the cerebral Trivial Pursuit— too easy to divide the room between smart and idiot. Games need to be one IQ point above Go Fetch.

Keep the attitude light and festive. Pour drinks, play the Party Mix music, distribute coasters, adjust the lighting, get the ashtrays and lighters if necessary. Avoid heated discussions over whether or not "she cheated, he peeked" or "that is too my goddam dollar!" The game is a means to an end, not an Olympic event.

Dice games are fun if they're simple. Card games that involve simple math or luck are fun. There is a book called *IF* and it has hundreds of questions you can ask a person about life, romance or sex. They are each under three separate titles. It can be fun if you pick a random number and the other person must read you a question from that page.

I cheated once. After twenty minutes of some adult questions like, "if you could have sex with somebody famous, who would it be?" I had her pick a number, I turned to the page, and then made up a question: "If you had to have a three way with any one of your friends, who would it be?" She rolled her eyes for a split second and said, "definitely Michelle."

"Why?" I asked.

"Because she's gorgeous and has a perfect body."
I pressed it further by asking what was perfect and I believe she used the words "breasts, butt and legs" in close succession.

There you have it: we have the same taste in women. The game revealed what would have otherwise been privileged information. Now I don't feel out of line suggesting a trip to the Jacuzzi.

Finally, playing a game should be a spontaneous suggestion, not a way to get people to your house.

- → Never say, "Who wants to come over and play a board game based on Delaware's shitty economy?"
- → Never suggest an obscure card game: "You guys wanna go back to my pad and play 9-card Pumpernickel?"
- → Never suggest a game that requires a permit or special shoes.

After a while, people lose interest in the game and, after a few cocktails, all they want to do is see how far they can throw the pieces or see whether the dice will float in a shot glass.

Player's love to play and that includes billiards, poker, craps, darts, and blackjack. But by now you've outgrown "quarters," Nintendo and duck, duck, goose. James Bond never played Marco Polo in the swimming pool with a beautiful Russian spy.

HIDE THE EVIDENCE

Player's Rule

Clean up after yourself

A woman may have a hunch that you're A Player, but you don't need to throw it in her face. Let her live with her suspicions; don't leave anything lying around that removes all doubt. It's okay to be a ladies man. It's even okay to be a "bad boy." That's why male celebrities who throw a couch out a hotel window, get in fist fights with photographers, and check in for rehab are in big demand. Women are intrigued, mildly aroused and feel "safe" in the company of a dangerous guy who shows her affection. Guys on death row get love letters everyday. OJ Simpson still gets laid. But keep obvious signs of steady traffic at your house on the down-low.

Beware of the following:

→ Lipstick on the end of cigarette butts
→ Lipstick on the rim of a wine glass
→ Condoms in the trash
→ Small pieces of the foil condom wrapper on the floor
→ Stains on the sheets
→ Earrings and their tiny backings
→ Her sunglasses
→ Eyeliner on your white towels
→ Tampon packaging
→ Rings

- → Her business card laying around
- → Contact lens wash if you don't wear contacts
- → Phone numbers on cocktail napkins
- → Panties stapled to the bulletin board in the kitchen
- → Lip balm with an applicator
- → Anything girly-girl a tough guy like you can't explain

Here's a stupid move I made before I earned my Player's stripes. I was returning from the kitchen with a couple of beers and saw something on the carpet. I handed her a beer and said, "Hey, you dropped something." I proudly handed her the earring as if I'd returned a lost puppy. She looked at it as if it were bad meat. "This isn't mine," she stated. I blamed it on the housekeeper (see chapter).

Women want to feel special, although they know you have six other days of the week to ply your trade. Be meticulous about removing all the evidence that you've had other company—if they see evidence, it's a major turn off. Play it cool, and create a "blank slate" at your house, free from all signs of last night's good time, and you can't get hurt.

THE JACUZZI AND THE POOL

Player's Rule

The Jacuzzi and the pool are a secret until she sees it

I've lost a few deals here. You get so excited at the prospect of getting her back to your house and in the water that you mention it as a selling point. "Hey listen, why you don't and your friends join us for a little Jacuzzi party later? It's a great night for it." If they've seen the pool or Jacuzzi, you have a chance. If they're new contacts, it will scare them away.

If you're a woman, what comes to mind when you think of late night water sports? The following:

- → "I don't have a bathing suit"
- → "I'm not shaven down there"
- → "Panties, bras, nudity"
- → "Debbie's on her period"
- → "I'll catch a cold"
- → "I don't want people to see my scar"
- → "I don't want people to see my tattoo"
- → "My ass is out of shape"
- → "I'm so white this time of year"
- → "I have a bruise on my lower back from screwing last night"
- → "I can't get naked in front of my coworkers"

I've had exceptions where the girls say, "Great! Let's go!" But for the most part, asking them over to the pool is tantamount to asking them to remove their clothing on the spot. Asking too soon will make them sense your direct agenda.

Better to have them over for another reason, and then let them see the pool and give them the old, "coulda hadda V-8" look, and suggest it then. Just ask, "Who's in for a dip in the pool?" Sometimes it's fun to assume the sale, drop your pants and jump in. If they want to change clothes, offer a short, white t-shirt.

HIDE THE PORN

Player's Rule

Keep porn out of sight

I knew guys who thought they were cool, or exercising their right to be a male, by leaving a skin magazine in plain view, or channel surf and stop when they see a man mounting two women on the hood of a car. Porn is like farting: it's something we enjoy *privately*.

Never, ever have a "toy" around that she didn't purchase *with you*. If you reveal a vibrator or handcuffs, she'll cringe at the hygiene violation. Unless you pay for it with her, and she removes it from the package *personally*, she's gonna freak. It's the equivalent of handing her a pair of panties you found under a hotel bed and asking her to try them on for size.

NO MEANS NO

Player's Rule

No means no

This is easy to use if you get a conditional "no." That's when they say, "Okay, I'll go with you, but that doesn't mean I'm sleeping with you!" This means "I'm interested in sleeping with you, but I haven't made up my mind yet." All you did was suggest another bar and her mind jumped to sex. Either way, you must honor her wishes. A Player is a gentleman with a strategy.

When they tell you it's platonic, or they've drawn boundaries, agree with them. Tell them, "No problem, we can have fun without getting crazy." Act as if she said, "I'd like to go to your house, but you can't give me an enema." Okay, whatever. It's the last thing that crossed your mind. This will concern her. When her attitude says, "I really can't," your attitude should say, "I don't give a shit."

When a woman draws the line, they think they canceled Christmas. They feel like they pulled the prize out of reach. They're waiting for a reaction since they feel they have all the control. They may shed a crocodile tear as they proceed to ruin your evening, so fight fire with fire. When you pretend to be totally unaffected, they become self-conscious. She'll wonder if it's her gingivitis or if you noticed her third nipple. As soon as you act like you don't care, change the subject: "Did Dallas win the game tonight?" Mention a beautiful girl you were madly in love with two years ago. Tell her what you loved about her and make sure the one you're with has *none* of those traits.

If the woman I'm with is short with brown eyes, I tell her this story: "I mean she was great. She had a smile that would stop traffic, long legs, big blue eyes—like looking at a swimming pool—and what a body." Then appear to snap out of your daydream: "Anyway, you only get those once in a lifetime—so where did you say you went to college?" As she tries to remember, she's looking down at her piano bench legs with her brown eyes. "He can't possibly find me attractive" is screaming in her brain.

If I'm with a blonde who's happy to drink my money but isn't sure if I'm worth kissing, I pull the same stunt. I somehow mention the fact that I love Latin women—"Their striking, raven hair and their passion for everything. They really know how to treat a man." And then change the subject: "By the way, I get free text messaging after two in the morning."

Women want what they can't have and when they perceive that they have no control over you, they slowly begin to play the game. They'll return from the ladies room with their panties in their purse if they have to. Your indifference wipes the slate clean and you still have a shot at romance.

SNOOPING

Player's Rule

Don't snoop

You're seated in your living room and she asks to use your bathroom. When she leaves, it's you, the candle and the stereo—and her purse. You stare at the purse and you hear the toilet seat drop. This gives you five minutes, tops.

You're tempted to peek inside her purse. Who called her cell phone? Let's see the picture on her driver's license. How much does she weigh? Don't do it. If anything, you'll find something that turns you off. It's never worth getting caught and if she weighs eight pounds more than she said, you still want to see her naked. Worst case scenario: you return her wallet to the purse upside down and she'll know you snooped. She'll wonder how much cash is missing.

If you use her bathroom, don't snoop. She can hear the medicine cabinet magnets kissing a half a mile away. You'll only find disturbing little bottles. Every drug you find will sound like a leprosy inhibitor.

The one time I did look in a girl's medicine cabinet, I was horrified. I read labels as fast as my eyes could eat the words. I was bludgeoned by a sea of medicinal words that made my mind reel: cream, ointment, salve, "one tablet daily," lots of amber bottles with serious white labels. There were applicators and Q-tips I could only put in the crudest of contexts. I saw pads and liners. There were at least two things I couldn't pronounce that had a "doxy" and a "phenyl-phosphate" on the label. I was certain she had only six months to live. My imagination made her toothpaste sound like a cure for flakey thighs.

It's okay if *you* get a pimple or athlete's foot, but a woman with Gas-x or Preparation-H should carry a little bell around the house. Ignorance is bliss.

GETTING RID OF THE OVERNIGHT GUEST

Player's Rule

You always have stuff to do the next day

I never say anything about my agenda until after the deal is closed. If they ask me about my next day, I tell them I have a few things going on and then ask them some unrelated question: "What's the state motto of Vermont?" I want them to think I'm worry-free at night. In the morning, I want them to believe I'm late for a meeting. After all, A Player is very serious about his career.

Don't get me wrong, if you want to cuddle the following morning until noon, go for it. But if you need to gracefully get on with your life, here are a few tactics: After you've had your fun, ask her about her next day. Whatever she says, tell her about your meeting the following morning. If it's a weekend, tell her about the oddball family thing you're dreading. Once you've planted the seed, you may now retire assured that you can get up and start your day with a sense of urgency. Finally, prepare with a few additional details.

Set the alarm clock and program your coffee maker. When you get up, shave or shower or whatever is fitting for the "occasion." Be nice, be cordial, be sweet, and be focused. Ask her if you can pour her a quick cup of coffee. Eventually you walk her to her car or—for you New Yorkers—to the elevator of the building—give her a kiss and tell her you'll call her later in the afternoon.

I've actually walked a girl to her car and driven off in my car only to circle the block, stop at Starbuck's, and then return home to my peaceful sanctuary. Now I'm free to relax, catch some sports, scratch, and make a sandwich. This may seem insensitive but it's better for people who appreciate privacy. She can take her time in the shower and you can fart freely.

The key is *compassion*. You need to make this happen without her feeling slighted. It's not that you don't like her, but there's no point in allowing breakfast to snowball into a day at the museum.

PET NAMES

Player's Rule

A single pet name speaks volumes

Never has so much been made of a single word or phrase like a pet name. I worry when I'm at dinner and she passes me the olive oil and says, "Here you go, sweetie." Sweetie is the equivalent of "exclusive" and "monogamous." This may be good news. She likes you. "Sweetie, babe, and honey," are terms of endearment. The subtext is, "I like you, I like your company, and I will throw a shit fit if I catch you with another woman after I screwed you silly this weekend." Be careful not to use a pet name yourself unless you're hanging up those golden gloves.

Other Pet Names

Women are players, too. They'll read this book so they know what you're thinking. Their dating schedule is busier than yours. They can go out every night and play the game; here's why:

→ The men pay so it's free.
→ They don't have to sleep with him, so even their period is not an obstacle.
→ They are multi-orgasmic and some try to maximize this gift.
→ They never need Viagra.
→ They hide beneath the guise of trying to find Mr. Right.

News flash: They are juggling dates and men if they answer the phone with

→ Hey you!
→ Hey sweetie!
→ Hi handsome!
→ What's up?
→ What's happening?
→ What's the word humming bird?

These are fronts that prevent the potential for blurting the wrong name or trying to remember and stammering.

Although I don't recommend snooping, I did open a girlfriend's cell phone once and scrolled through the names in her database. It was packed with guys' names, not to mention names like T-bone and Sully. That's a lot of dudes for a girl with one sister and no boyfriends.

When I called her and she answered the phone with a big "Hey you," I knew she wasn't sure if it was me or T-bone. When she later told me she's out with friends and using the ladies room, I knew she was A Player. If she's with friends, there's nothing wrong with making a two-second phone call from the table. If she's with a guy, she needs to call as fast as she can pee and wash her hands. Divest yourself of this multi-tasker because she's less sincere than you—and probably T-Bone.

DAMAGE CONTROL

Player's Rule

Covering your bases is a class move

What do you do if you had a big night with a woman, and decided she's not a candidate for your next girlfriend? Damage control.

Damage control is best defined as a chivalrous way to phase out a relationship before you get in too deep. It's a time where you can be kind, pleasant and fair, and somewhat unavailable. If you fail to do some kind of damage control, you will burn a bridge.

Damage control is best executed from a cell phone. Cell phones have just enough poor reception to mask subtleties in your tone; and cell phones give the impression that you are a busy person on-the-go. If you call from your car with the window cracked, you will provide the ambient noise required to sound like a man on his way to the airport. This may sound insensitive, but it is the lesser of two evils. If you never call, it's worse and they will not forgive you. If you are simply inaccessible for a while, the flame blows out on its own.

Here's what to say:

"Hi (Lisa) it's Johnny, how goes it? Just calling to say I had fun last night—thanks for the (cocktails and all the fun); I'm out today taking care of business before my week from hell starts. Catch up with me later . . . talk to you then. Bye."

I like to call before noon the following day which shows you care, and then you can relax the rest of the day having satisfied her emotions. A Player always wants to remain in good standing with his female friends.

Text messaging or emailing is transparent. You might as well hide behind a tree and have your friend break up with her for you. Damage control is rarely achieved with any credibility unless they hear a voice.

You are not *obligated* to take a woman to dinner on a "real date" just because you slept with her the first time you met her any more than she is *obligated* to pay for you or sleep with you on the first date because you took her to dinner. You both shared an evening of mutual value and you both have the right to advance or retreat.

NOW WHAT?

Player's Rule

It's a process, not an event

Congratulations! You finished a manual that will improve your odds at romance immediately. Here are a few things to keep in mind:

→ These skills must be applied in order to work
→ If applied, they will improve the situation
→ You will become "fluent" with these ideas the more you practice
→ Adopt these skills and deliver them in your own style
→ Sometimes they don't work, but that's the exception

Yes, even the best of us Players use a basic tactic and it falls flat. Don't panic. It's like betting on blackjack in Vegas. Sometimes you're handed a pair of Kings and the dealer shows a 6 but still lands a 21. What happened? Nothing; you had a great advantage, did what the "book" recommends, but sometimes "it's not in the cards." Get back on your horse and continue with my correct strategy.

Have fun with my ideas. See you out on the town!

Cheers!

The Player

APPENDIX

More things every player should know

Conversation and Body Language

Many people just ignore the necessity of developing the fine art of conversation and take it for granted that it doesn't matter how you carry it out as long as the others involved in the conversation understand what you are saying. That is the main reason why we hear crude and vulgar language often used in conversation. It is also true that most conversations are just empty gossip without constructive content. It may be all right if you are just passing your time over a cup of coffee in a coffee shop with some friends who wouldn't care a dime about what is happening and where it happens.

I am sure you must have the experience of engaging in an interesting conversation for hours on end and yet you do not realize it has taken that long. You are so engrossed in the conversation that you sometimes even forget an important appointment. Likewise, you may have also joined in a conversation and are very anxious to get out of it as the topics become dull and boring. That being said, I am also now sure that you know the reasons why in one instance you are so engrossed while at another you want to leave at the first opportunity.

Conversation is an art that must be mastered if you want to be successful with your audience, if you want people to pay attention to you and keep them glued to their seats. In this seduction exercise, a mastery of the art of conversation is a must if you want your partner glued to her seat paying attention to every word you say.

The first rule is to respect the woman, to speak less and listen more. God gave us one mouth and two ears for a reason. Remember the rule, that a social conversation is a conversation and nothing more. It is a two way process if you are alone with the woman, and a multi-involvement process if you are among friends. Right from the outset, you must refrain yourself from turning the conversation into a Sunday sermon or a debating platform or a political arena. These are the common blunders committed by many people who are easily carried away by the slightest provocation that suddenly and unexpectedly arises.

During the course of the conversation, sometimes sensitive issues arise that challenge your ego. Do not respond negatively to that. Be proactive; view the situation and suggestions or provocations from the other side of the coin, not from the usual antagonistic side. You may see some arguments that you can agree to. Stay cool and calm. Show that in your body language. Do not react, become fidgety and nervous, or unduly provoked and anxious to fight back. The attitude will look too childish and amateurish and will not speak much of your personality. Learn to see other people's view in parallel and do not impose a stoic and purely judgmental standard of 'there is one right' and all others are therefore wrong.

Just like you, other people too have their points of view, their assessments and judgments of the various phenomena around. Be gracious and accept their points of view proactively and in parallel to yours. This will not irritate them and soon they will be ever welcome to your presence.

During the course of every conversation, display the relaxed and comfortable stance of the alpha man. Smile occasionally when something interesting is being said but do not be eager to interrupt and chip in your piece in the subject. You must know when you are welcome to chip in to the conversation. Do not be over anxious to display your knowledge and show that you are more knowledgeable in all subjects well above and over the rest.

Don't get too cocky and believe people will admire you for your high intelligence. Please be warned that, exhibiting your knowledge at the wrong time and at the wrong place can do more harm than good. In a conversation, unlike in a debate, everybody wants to feel good and would be annoyed if you drive them into the back seat, and make them feel inferior in the eyes of others.

To add insult to injury, in your eagerness to show, there is a very strong tendency to step on the toes of others. There is also a tendency to highlight their stupidity through your tone of voice and body language. If you do that you will definitely break the camel's back and they will disappear one by one from the scene until you find yourself alone— talking to the wall like a lunatic.

When with the woman, just engage in light conversation, taking the cue from the key words she includes in her conversation. If you pay attention closely, you will know what interests her and what topics of conversation is natural to her. Take the cue from there and flow with the conversation. Should you come to terms that she uses and you are not sure what they mean, you can graciously apologize to her and ask for the meaning.

It would not be an exhibition of ignorance but you will be passing to her a powerful message that you are paying attention to what she is saying. She will appreciate that and conclude that you are a good conversation partner. Turn the conversation into an occasion of joy, devoid of all the trappings of an argument, debate or Sunday sermon.

Now when it is your turn to chip in, what are the suitable topics that you can bring in to make it interesting to the woman? It need not be of things that interest women and be about topics of conversations they have among themselves. You can narrate incidents that have a funny twist that happened maybe, during your fishing trip, or visit to an island or during your stay at an island resort. Chances are she might want to hear more, if the incident is similar to the ones she had experienced at one time or another before. If she shows eagerness to relate similar incidents of her own experience, take the opportunity to pass the helm to her. Use your body language to show your attentiveness and excitement about the phenomena while comparing its similarity to the one you experienced.

Indulging in a conversion about topics of common interests or common experience is always exciting and fun. It might draw a few giggles and light laughter. If that were to happen, don't hold back. By all means laugh. If she were the one who create the joke, she would be flattered. You can chip in with a similar joke if you like. It would make the encounter even more interesting. Whichever it is, make the conversation as natural and interesting as possible. An air of arrogance, know it all or undue show of superiority is definitely and strongly out of order.

Be gracious without being superficial or unnatural. Be cool, calm and collected without being dumb and uninteresting. If your presence adds color to many a dull conversation and if your contributions make it interesting and joyous, you can bet your last dollar that people will always look forward to having you in their conversational encounters.

If you have made a lasting impact and handled your conversation well, people will find that something is missing without you at the table or in the room. They might even invite you to join them for lunch, just listen to you and enjoy your fascinating company.

In a conversation, when you are saying something or are trying to put forward a point, your body language speaks volumes about you and the sincerity of your statements. The truth is usually spoken in a relaxed, non-fidgety way. The statements are rather casual yet convincing, expressed in stance of self-confidence. Once stated it is not repeated unless requested.

Statements presented in a jumbled up manner and with a nervous stance are seldom taken seriously. For one thing, people hearing you will not have a clue to what you are saying. For another, your voice and body language quickly gives you away as some moron who does not know what he is talking about and is juggling unfounded gossip to make it sound real.

How to Satisfy Your Lady in Bed

Sexuality is an important part of our lives. The desire to love, to give and receive intimacy and affection is integral to every successful relationship. Every man desires to be the alpha male who can win a woman's adoration and respect on and off the bed! When you talk about sex life, a true gentleman knows how to please his lady between the sheets. The way you made her feel in bed makes the whole world of difference between a fulfilling and joyous relationship and one that is heading towards the rocks!

We sometimes hear of women who choose to run away with another lover in spite of having everything else she needs. Often enough it has everything to do with her dissatisfaction with the way her man makes her feel in bed. Thus never disregard the ability to satisfy your lady as an important element to create a long lasting and enduring relationship.

Whether you are in a relationship in search of true meaningful love or merely for fun, the ability to satisfy your lady is an indispensable tool in the creation of the true gentleman.

How to Get Your First Kiss

If you have been paying attention, you should know by now that all women crave to be with a real man whom she can admire and look up to. Women do not want to be around little boys who whimper up and stutter.

The best way to get your first kiss with your woman is to watch her body language. Often you can see from her gestures what she really has in mind and wants. Try to be as close as possible to her. Make eye contact and watch her reaction. If she smiles and has a dreamy look in her eyes, chances are she wants to be kissed!

Lean towards her and give her soft gentle kiss on the lips and pull back. If she doesn't flinch or pull away, this time kiss her deeply and longer. The lips are the most erroneous zone and kissing her in the right way can drive her wild with passion. Now you are ready to explore further and take the relationship to the next level!

Learning the Most Intoxicating Kiss of All

French kisses are probably the most sensuous form of kissing in the world. A French kiss is where both partners use the tongues to explore the insides of your partner's mouth. It creates a thrilling and amazing sensation that will drive you and your partner wild with passion.

Before you start kissing your lady, make sure you have this checklist with you and ensure that you do not forget anything.

→ Make sure you have a clean mouth and clean white teeth. No one wants to be kissed by a bad breath male with unsightly teeth! Make regular visits to the dentist and floss your teeth on a regular basis.
→ Remember to relax when kissing your partner. A rigid body will give you away as an inept novice who is just learning to have the first kiss!
→ Open your lips to kiss her.

Get into a good position. If you place your face directly in front of her, your noses will bump into each other. Ideally, move it to one side so that your lips can reach each other comfortably.

Tongue Technique

Get your tongue inside your partners mouth an inch or two. Circle it around the tip of your lady's tongue. If she is doing something, you can follow her gesture and do accordingly. Respond to her tongue movements. Tongue technique involves flicking, exploring and light touching. The key is to keep your tongue moving inside her and do not stay still.

At this point, your lady should be ready to let you do your explorations further.

The Primary Erogenous Zones

Basically, women have two areas of erogenous zones: a primary and secondary zone. Here is the list of the primary erogenous zones that you want to access to turn her "buttons" on!

- → Mouth
- → Nipples
- → Breasts
- → Buttocks

Secondary Erogenous Zones

- → the nape of the neck
- → the small of the back
- → inside wrists
- → inside elbows
- → back of knees
- → thigh
- → feet

The way to turn her buttons is to start with her SECONDARY erogenous zones. Soft touches and caressing of her secondary erogenous zones can do miracles to make her ready for more.

When you see all the signs that are favorable move your caress to her primary erogenous zones. Kiss and fondle her breasts. Tweak those nipples. Kiss and fondle buttocks. Kiss her nipples then her breasts. Alternate and move very slowly. Play with all her primary erogenous zones.

Most women love to be teased so shower her with praises and tease her while you are at it.

When you finally reach her genitals place you lips on her clitoris and suck on it steadily. Use your tongue to freely lick around the clitoris in a circular motion. Do it slowly and steadily and this will bring about a powerful orgasm.

Cunnilingus

Cunnilingus is a form of foreplay that can bring a lady to levels of pleasure unknown before! In fact, cunnilingus can be considered sex without penetration. If initially, your lady is reluctant to have intercourse, this is the perfect way to satisfy her without pressuring with her for sex. Cunnilingus lets her enjoy the soft caress of your mouth without having to go all the way.

Before you start your explorations, there are some facts that you should keep in mind to ensure a smooth and pleasant journey.

Moist

Her private part consists of millions of nerve endings that are highly sensitive, so be sure to keep them moist before you start dabbling on them with your tongue. If you plan to insert any fingers into her, be sure those moist as well. Use your own saliva or hers. Any dry will pull on her skin and will be extremely uncomfortable for her.

Breathing and Body Movement

Her breathing and body movements can let you know her state of arousal at the moment. Sometimes, she may gasp for air or hold her breath. She may lie still, or heave about. The more response you get, the more your attempts to arouse her should continue.

Verbal Commands

Probably the most welcomed command that every gentleman wants to hear is the wonderful command, "Don't stop!" It means you are doing the right thing and you should not stop whatever you are doing!

When done correctly cunnilingus can give your lady a new form of enjoyment that will bring you closer together and share new heights of pleasure never known before.

Take it Slow

Women love to be pampered and caressed so do remember to take it very slow. Make her feel loved and wanted, and she will stick with you long after those lovemaking sessions are over.

Biggest Mistakes Men Make in Bed

Snore after Sex

After you've popped your cork, the worse thing you can do is to roll over and snore! Women hate the idea of being used just for their body, so be sure to caress her and whisper a soft loving word even AFTER sex so she will feel appreciated.

Premature Ejaculation

This is one of the most embarrassing things that can happen when you are making love to your lady. One or twice is considered normal, and you can explain it away by your amazement at your lady's beauty and sex appeal. However, if this happens every time, then you are in for some trouble. After all, if you fail to satisfy HER, why should she continue to have sex with you? If this occurrence occurs too many times, visit your doctor and get yourself some help.

Too Much of a Good Thing

If you have heard of multiple orgasms, do not misuse this to think that you have to make your lady orgasm for ten to fifteen times! If you make this your primary goal, chances are she will be so burnt out and you will never have a chance to touch her again for the next two weeks. Seriously prolonged sexual intercourse can cause a woman's delicate private parts to become irritated.

The Ten Commandments of Great Lovemaking

Take it Slow

Guys, remember that good sex isn't a race to see who finish first. The biggest pleasure for you may be the climax at the end, but for women there is pleasure all the while during the making of the course. So forget about the finishing fast if you really want to impress her.

Emotional Intimacy

Emotional intimacy is the essence to great lovemaking. Take time to share your desires and intimacies. Talk about what turns you on and what turns you off. Get her to open up and tell her about her own hot buttons as well.

Be Responsive

If you think going at it like a jackhammer is going to score you points with your lady, you are damn mistaken. Women do not relish the thought of a man who is out there solely for his own purpose. Learn to be responsive and sensitive to the lady's needs.

The Big 'O'

Very rarely do a woman orgasm through the penetration of the man's penis into her vagina. A woman's orgasm is more likely to come from stimulation to her most sensitive parts such as the clitoris—the bump located at the top of her vagina. So it takes a lot of yummy foreplay on your part.

Her Likes

If your lady doesn't know what she likes, then it is going to be difficult for you to figure out what to do to please her in bed. Ideally, encourage her to explore on her own and find out what are her own likes and dislikes.

Find the Right Moment

To have a great lovemaking session, find a nice time to get into the mood for love. If your lady is having a bad day or is tired after a hard days work, don't expect her to have a energetic time on the bed.

Exercise
Always make the effort to stay in shape. Maintain a good exercise routine. Both diet and exercise have a big influence on how you will perform in bed. If you want to make impression between the sheets, take the steps to inculcate a good exercise routine and maintain a healthy diet.

Don't Leave your Stomach Empty
Sex is undoubtedly a strenuous physical routine, so your body will need to draw upon its reserves of energy. Get yourself a nice supply of energy supplying carbohydrates such as pasta, rice, bread and such before you engage in such activities. It helps you to gain that extra energy without being burnt out prematurely.

Change Positions
Forget the missionary position as the only form of lovemaking. Get hold of a good sex guide books that will introduce you to a whole world of sexual positions that can amaze your partner. Vary the place and the time too. A little surprise here and there can do wonders to spice up your erotic journey.

Bring Romance
This is the magic word that can light up your lady's heart and mind. Women love romantic men who know how to treat a lady. Surprise her with love notes, flowers and thoughtful gifts. You will reap the rewards when you hit the sack.

Also Available from Tommy Orlando:

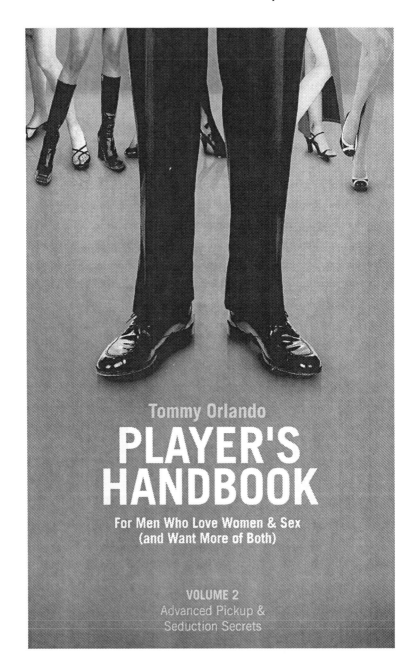

Tommy Orlando

PLAYER'S HANDBOOK

For Men Who Love Women & Sex
(and Want More of Both)

VOLUME 2
Advanced Pickup &
Seduction Secrets

Breinigsville, PA USA
15 April 2010
236259BV00004B/22/A